Wilson Tries New Foods

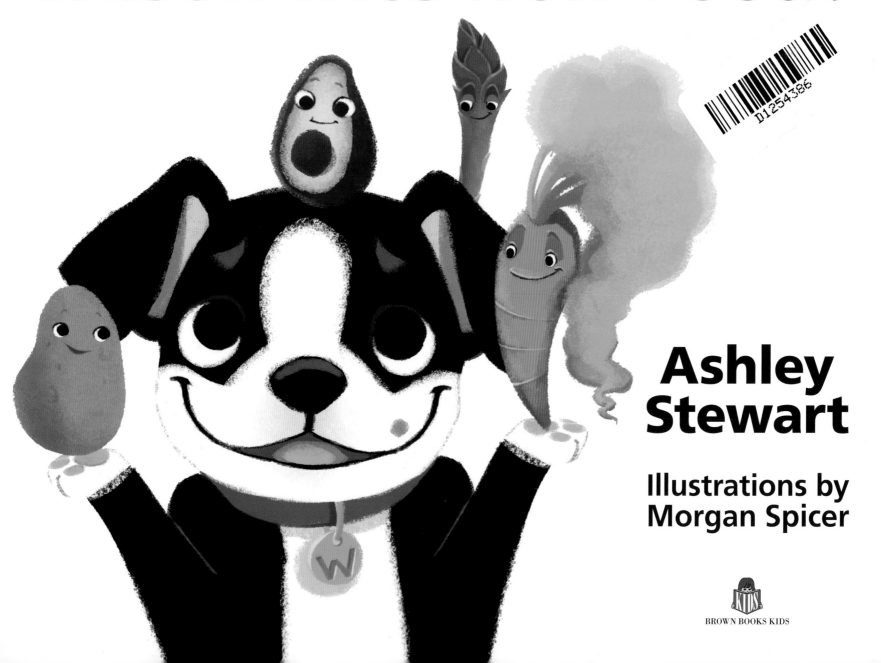

Ashley Stewart

Illustrations by
Morgan Spicer

BROWN BOOKS KIDS

The nutrition information provided in this book may differ from that of the Dietary Guidelines for Americans, developed jointly by the Department of Health and Human Services (HHS) and the United States Department of Agriculture (USDA). What you will find in this book is founded on Ashley Stewart's education, research, and both personal and professional experiences. Readers should perform their own research and consult with medical professionals before making significant changes to their diet and lifestyle.

Wilson Tries New Foods

Brown Books Kids
16250 Knoll Trail Drive, Suite 205
Dallas, Texas 75248
www.BrownBooksKids.com
(972) 381-0009

A New Era in Publishing™

ISBN 978-1-61254-228-7
LCCN 2014957747

Printed in the United States
10 9 8 7 6 5 4 3 2 1

For more information or to contact the author, please go to
www.EatWellWithWilson.com

Dedication
To Hadyn, Maddie, and Jack

Acknowledgments
Thank you to my family and friends for all of your support. I love you so much!

And special thanks goes to Earlene King, my longtime neighbor and dear friend. Your encouragement and contributions to this book are immeasurable. I could never have done it without you.

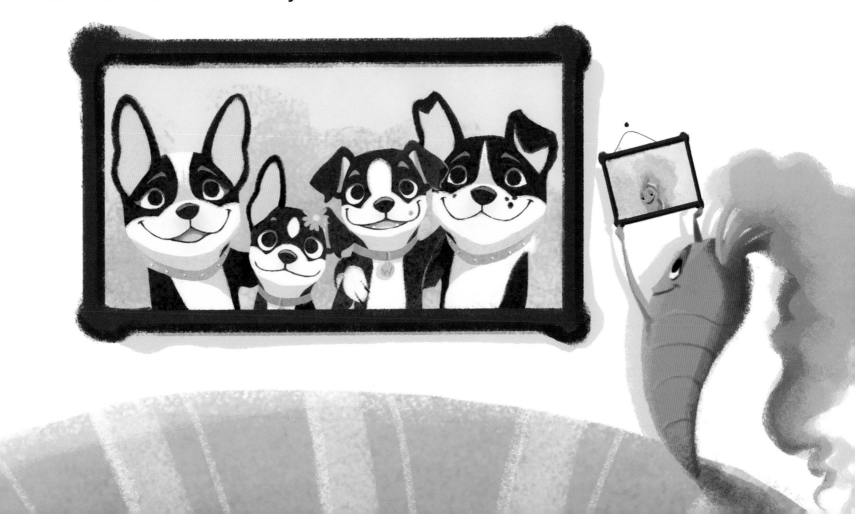

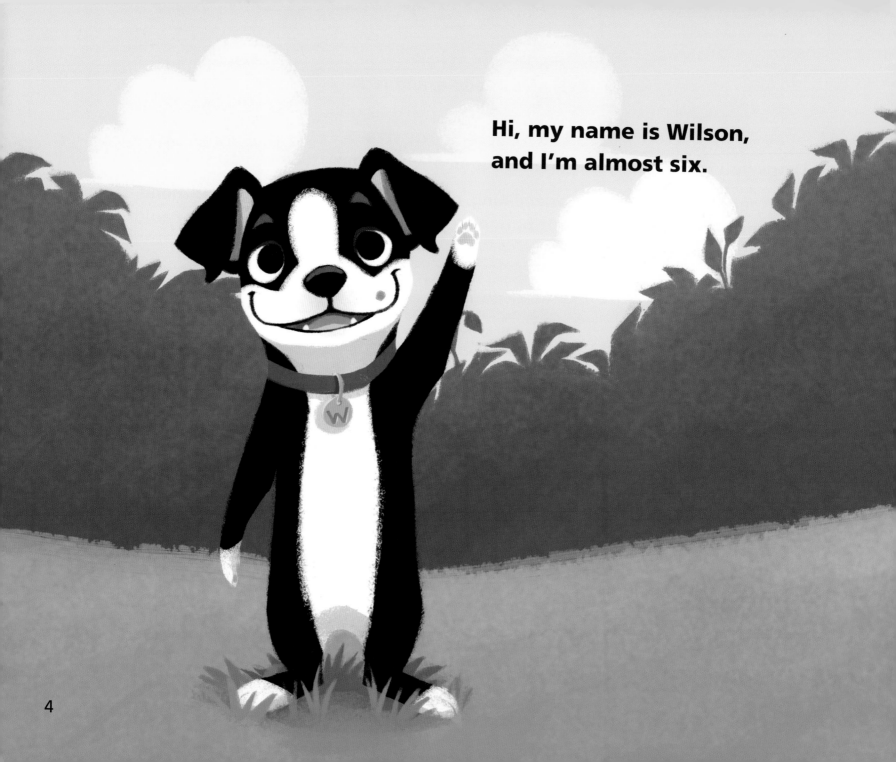

Hi, my name is Wilson,
and I'm almost six.

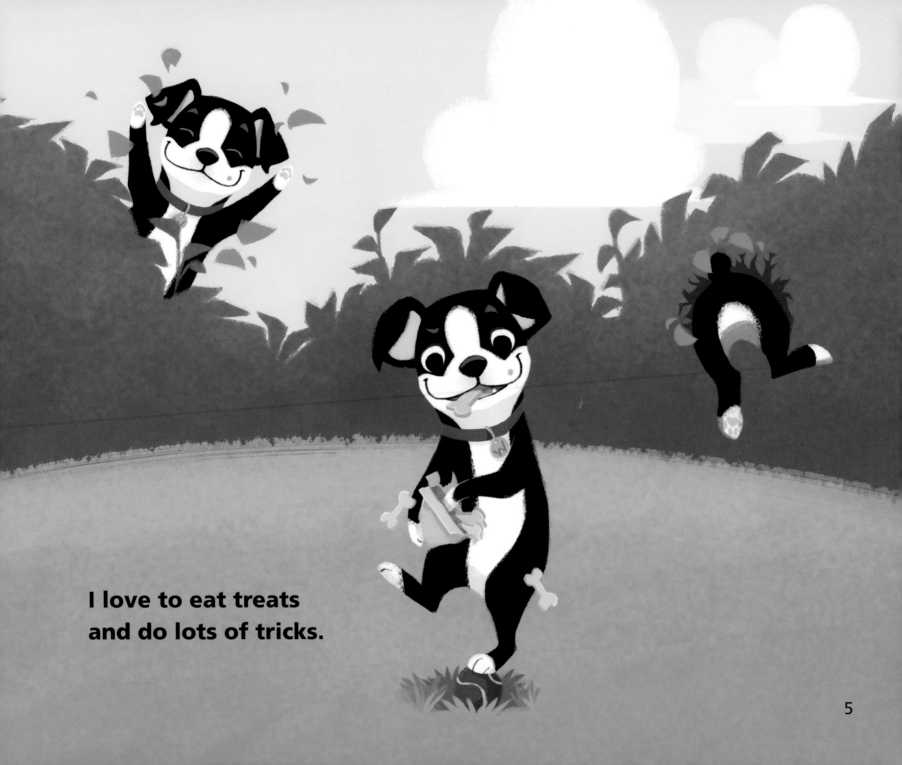

I love to eat treats
and do lots of tricks.

5

I have a little story that I want to tell
about an important day when I learned to eat well.

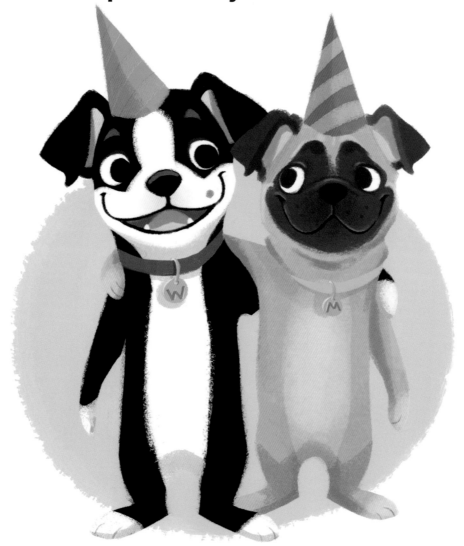

My story begins the day I went to a party.
It was a celebration for my best friend, Marty.

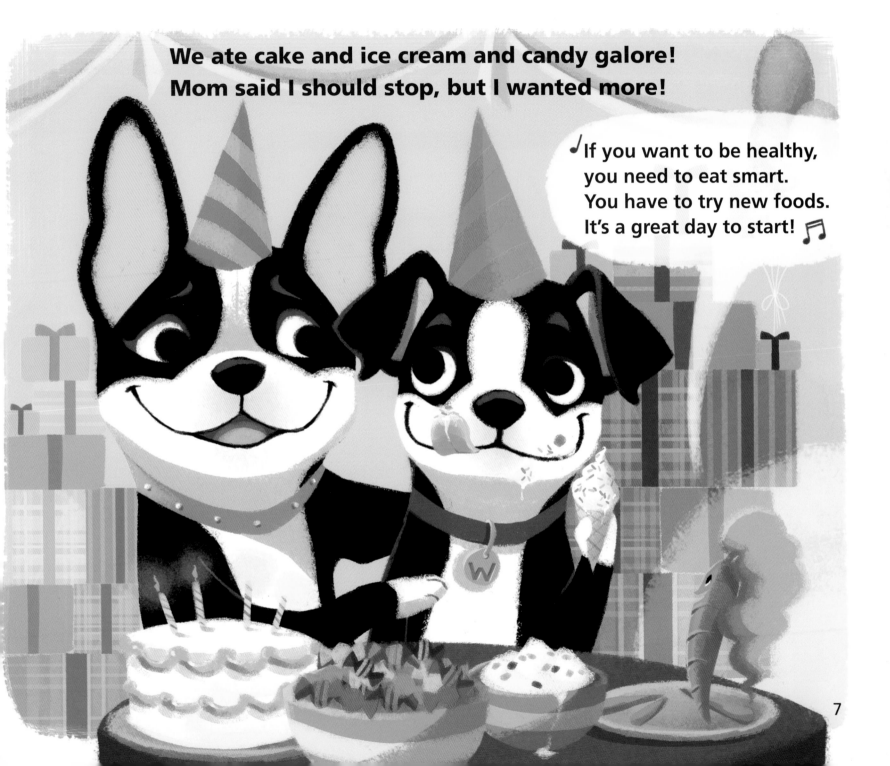

We ate cake and ice cream and candy galore!
Mom said I should stop, but I wanted more!

♪ If you want to be healthy,
you need to eat smart.
You have to try new foods.
It's a great day to start! ♫

7

Well, I was feeling great until the next day.
I was a GROUCH ON THE COUCH . . . as my mom would say.

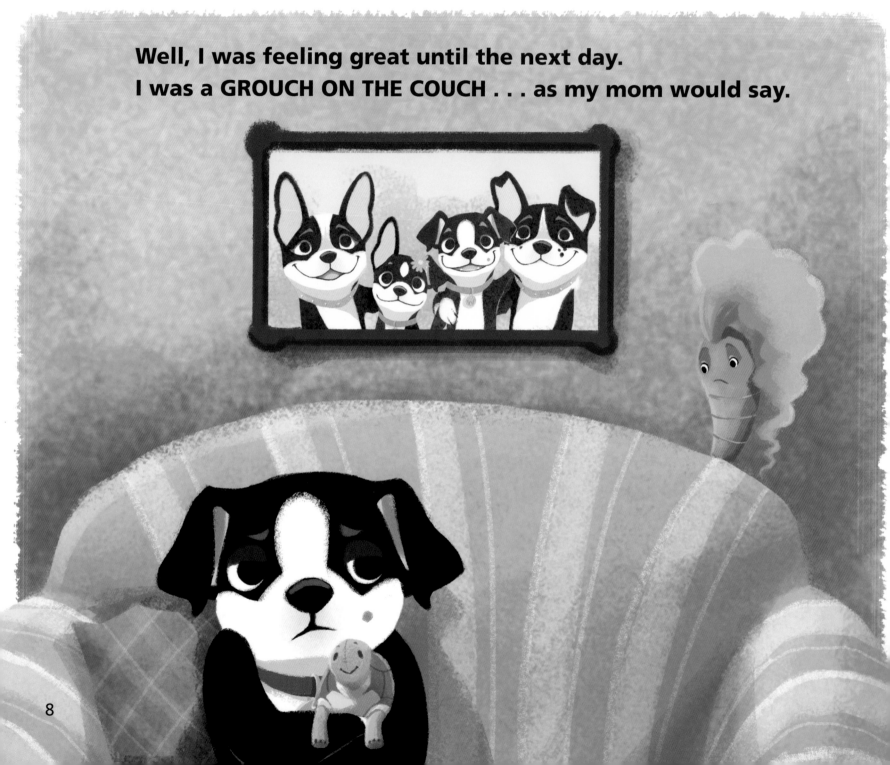

"What's wrong?" asked my mom. "Are you feeling crummy?"
"I'm in a bad mood," I whined. "It hurts in my tummy."

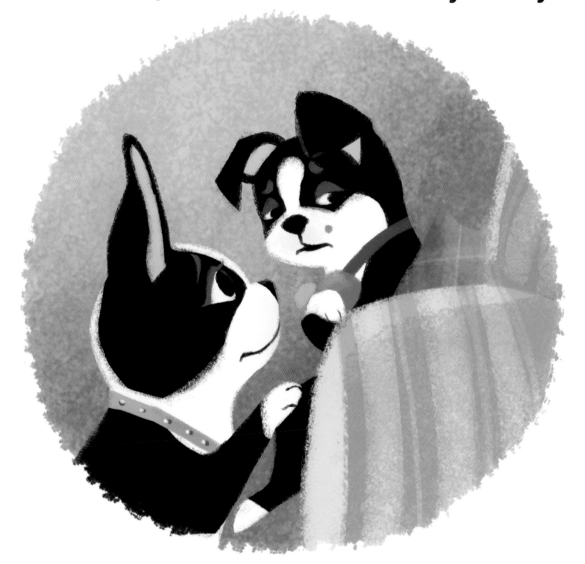

Then Mom calmly whispered, "Wilson, my sweet pet,
I think it's about time we visit the vet."

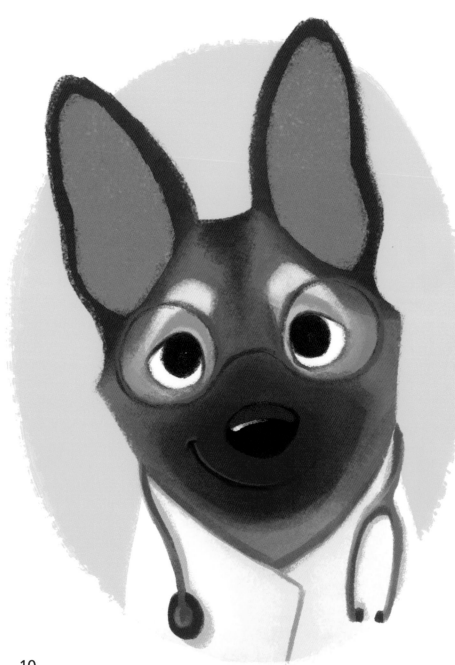

I love Doc Matthews.
He really is neat!
But he's always asking
about the food I eat.

When Doc saw me, he said,
"Wilson, you don't look so good.
Have you been eating
the way that you should?"

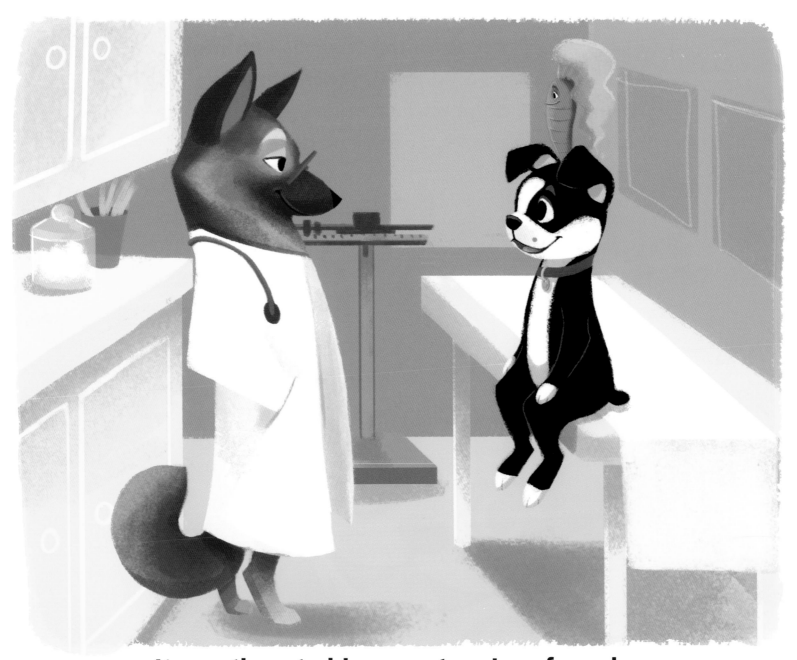

It was then, to him, my story I confessed.
"Well, maybe I haven't been eating my best."

"I was at a party with my friends last night.
The food was so yummy! It was out of sight!
We had hot dogs and chips and soda and cake!
I ate a huge piece . . . for goodness' sake!"

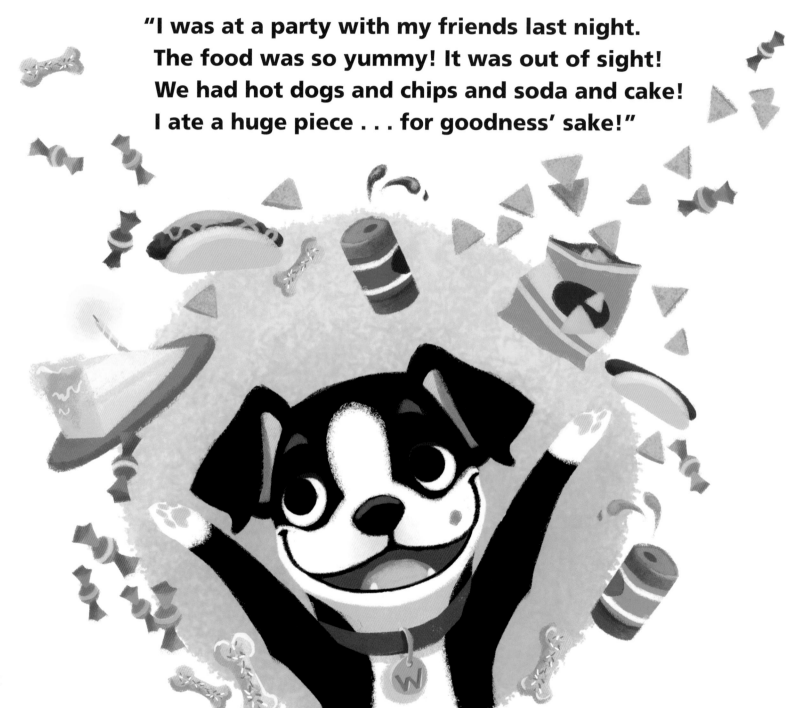

Doc exclaimed, "Oh no!
Watch out for sugar!
Inside our bodies,
it's a bad little booger.

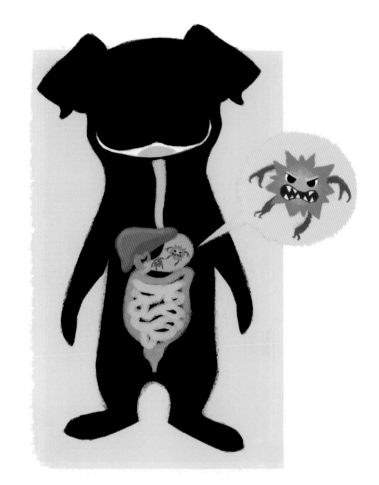

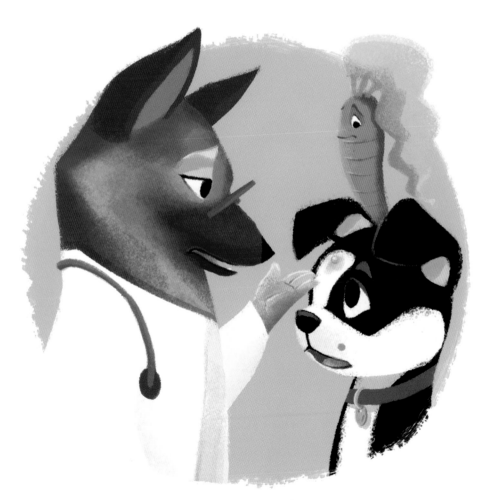

Sugar can make you feel
sick, tired, and grumpy.
Believe it or not,
it can make your face bumpy."

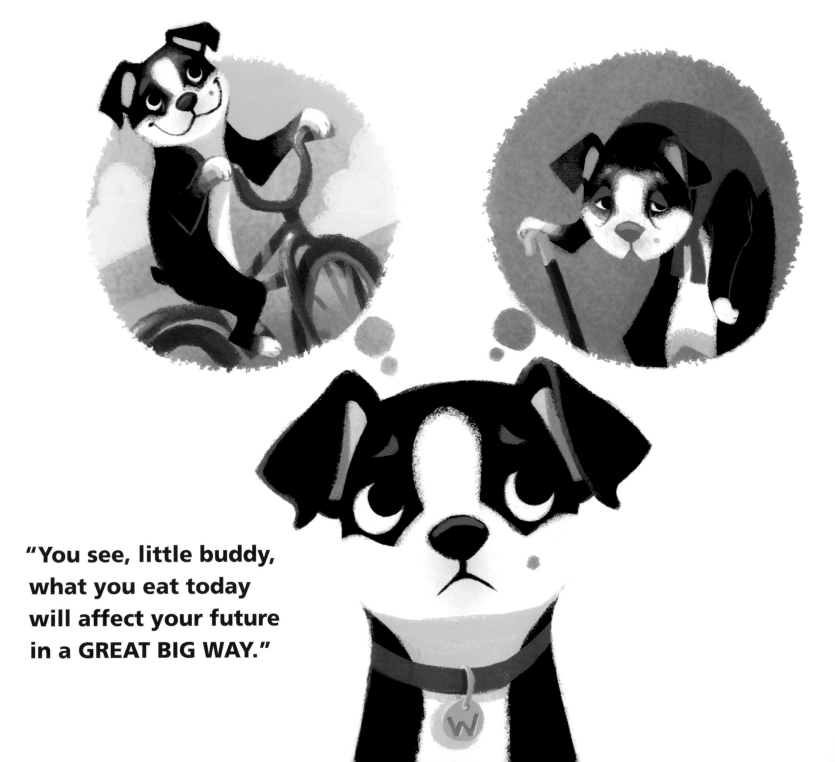

"You see, little buddy,
what you eat today
will affect your future
in a GREAT BIG WAY."

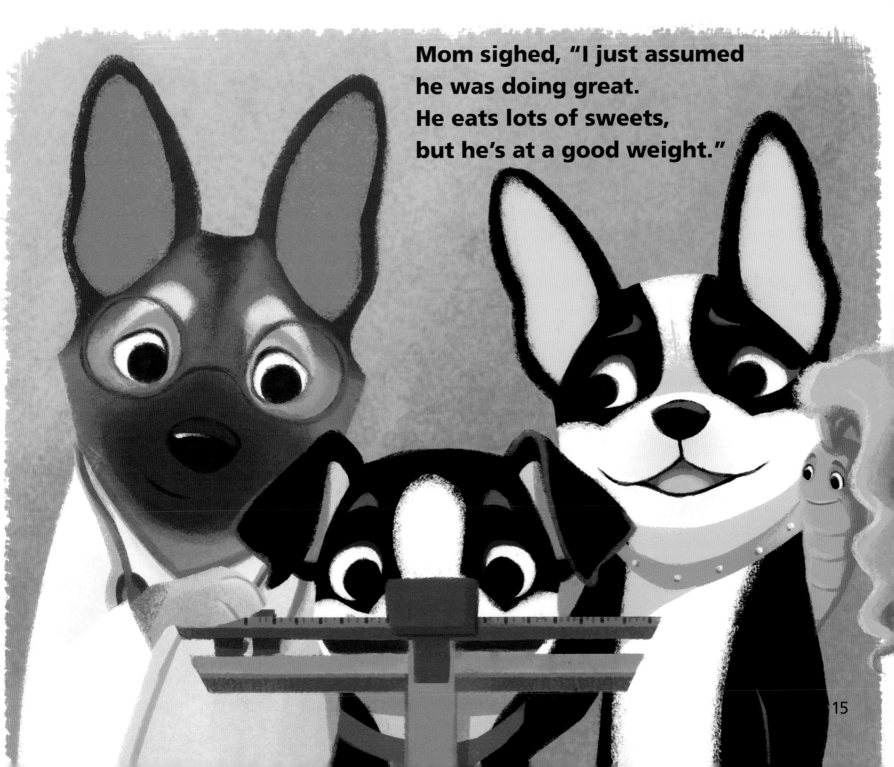

Mom sighed, "I just assumed
he was doing great.
He eats lots of sweets,
but he's at a good weight."

15

"You are right," said Doc. "His weight is just fine, but weight can be misleading. Look at these patients of mine."

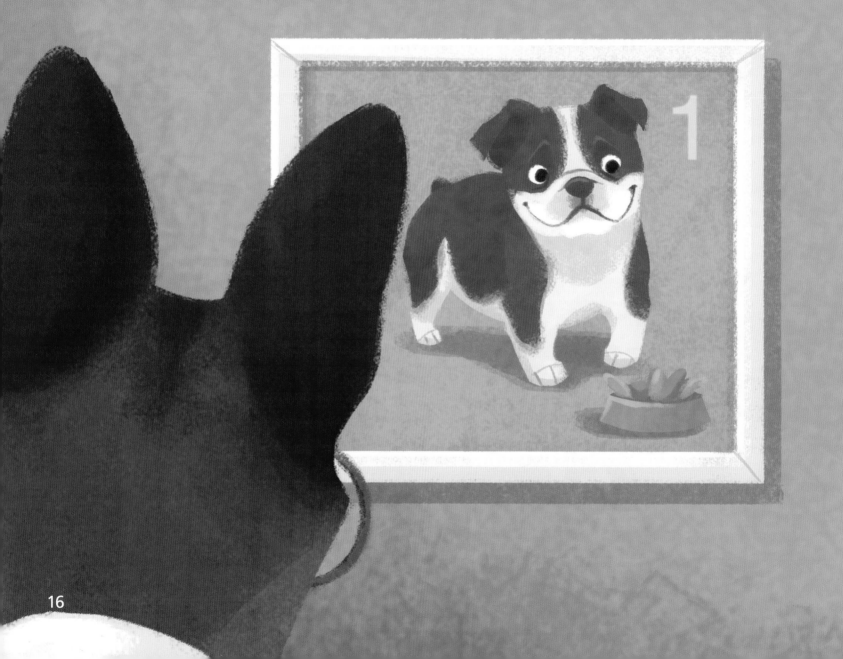

"We come in all sizes, some big and some small,
but poor nutrition can affect us all."

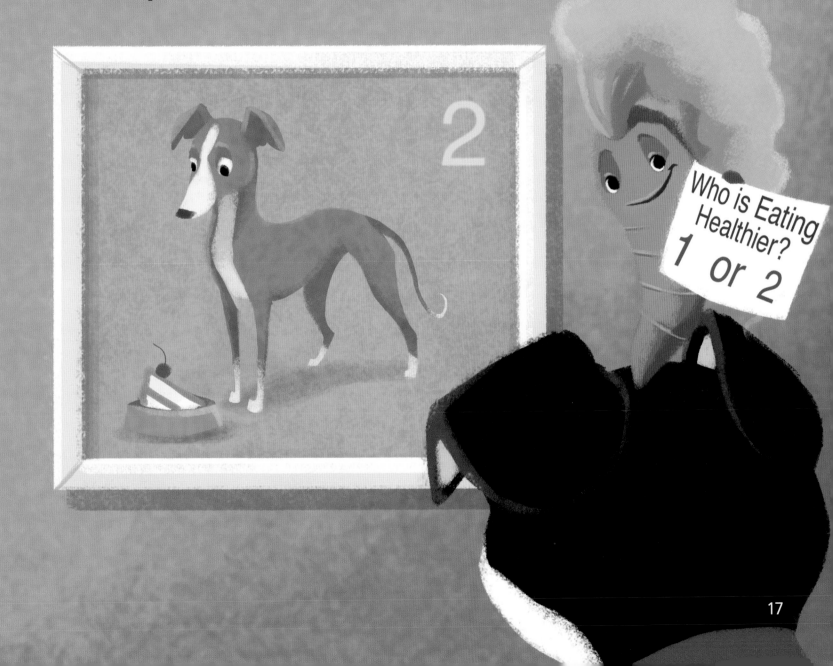

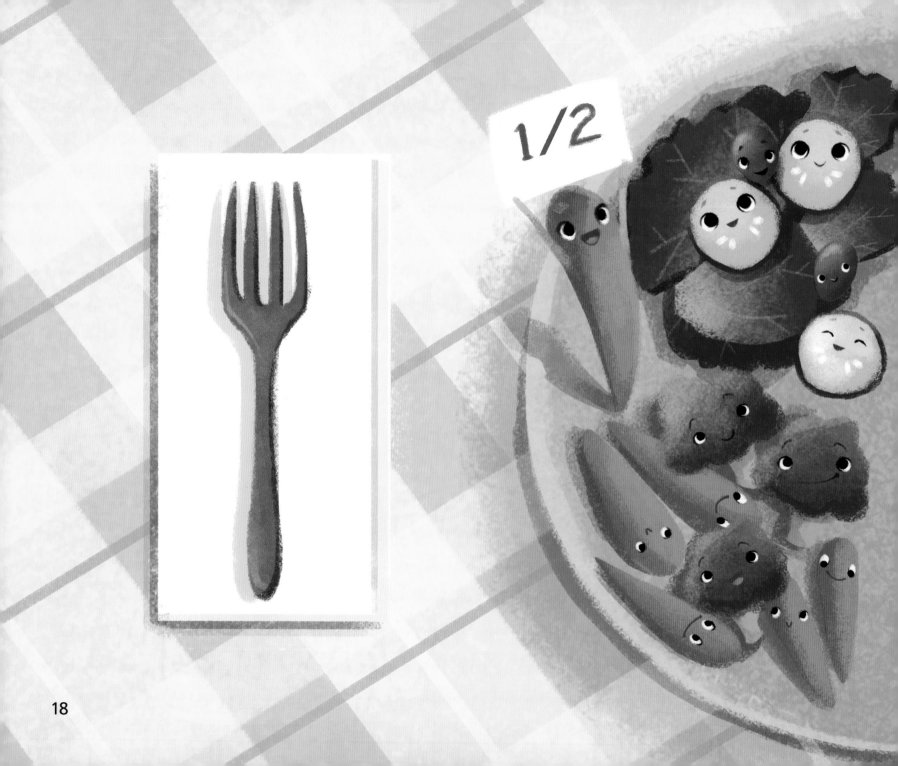

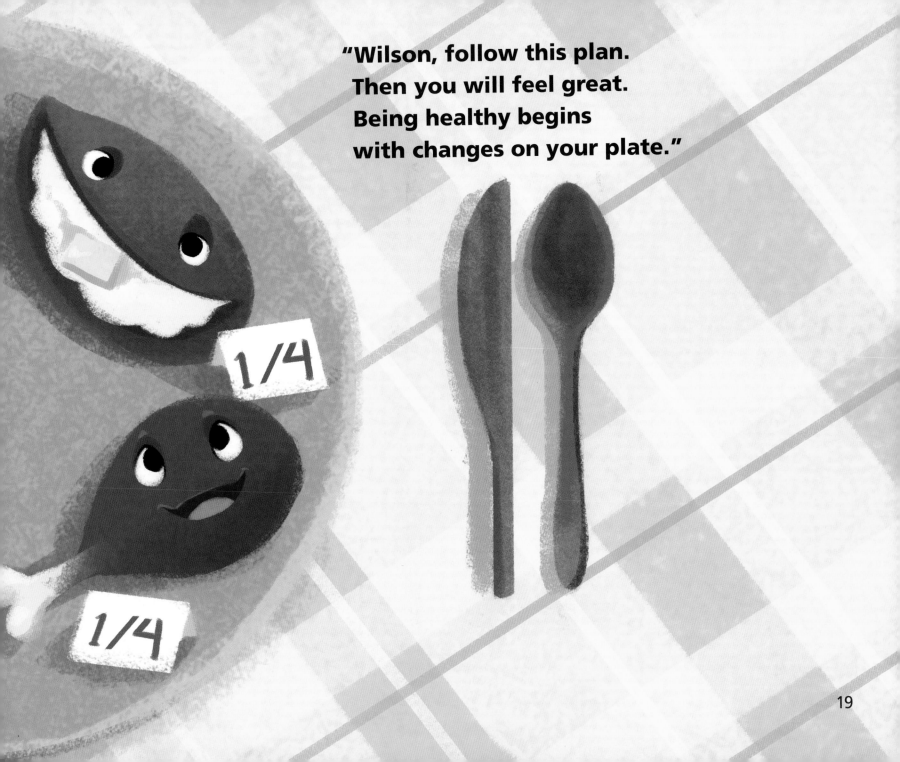

"Wilson, follow this plan.
Then you will feel great.
Being healthy begins
with changes on your plate."

1/4

1/4

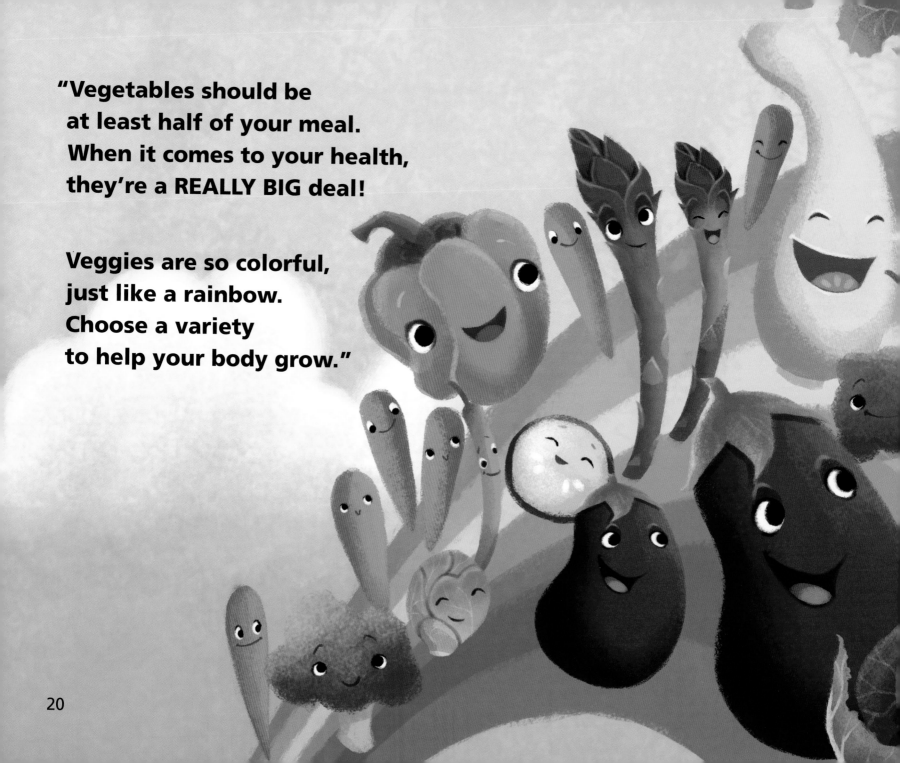

"Vegetables should be
at least half of your meal.
When it comes to your health,
they're a REALLY BIG deal!

Veggies are so colorful,
just like a rainbow.
Choose a variety
to help your body grow."

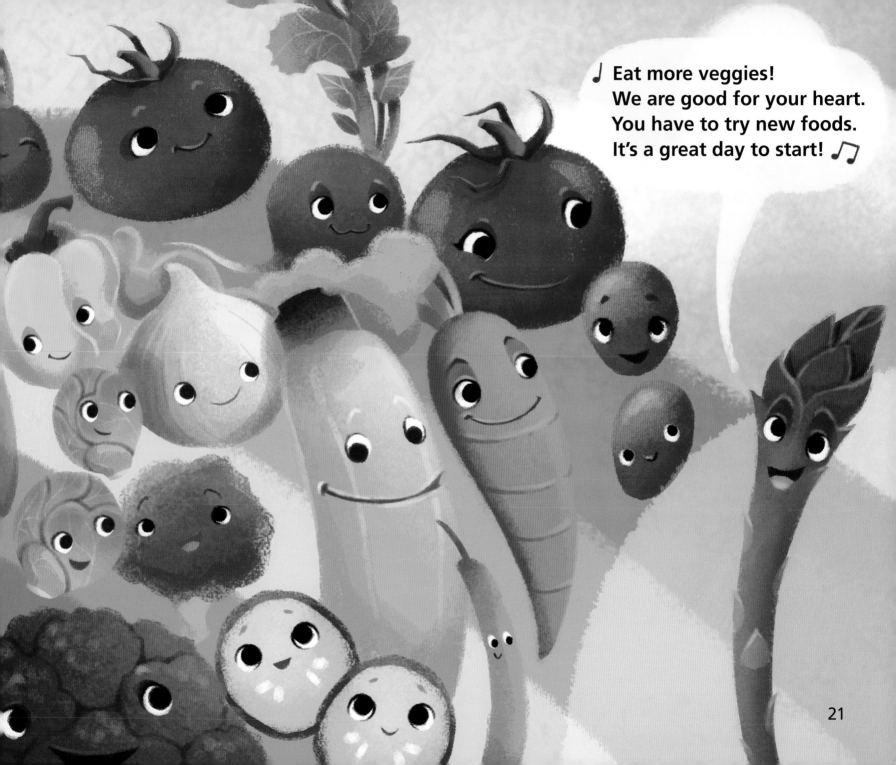

♪ Eat more veggies!
We are good for your heart.
You have to try new foods.
It's a great day to start! ♫

21

"Wilson, this next food group
will keep you strong and lean.
Can you guess what it is?
You're right! It's protein!

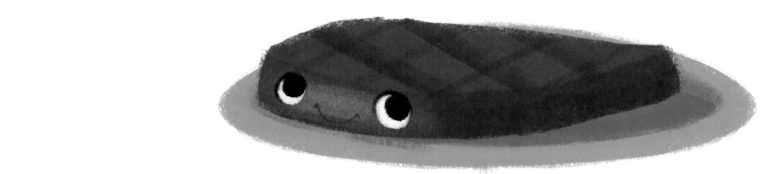

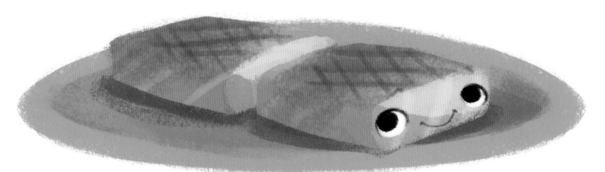

Protein includes foods
like beef, poultry, or fish.
But you can choose other
things if you wish."

"You might like pork, eggs, wild game, nuts, or cheese. It's great for you to eat healthy foods like these."

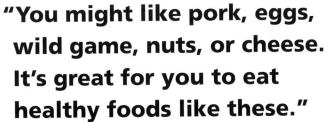

♫ We can help you grow strong. We're glad to do our part. You have to try new foods. It's a great day to start! ♫

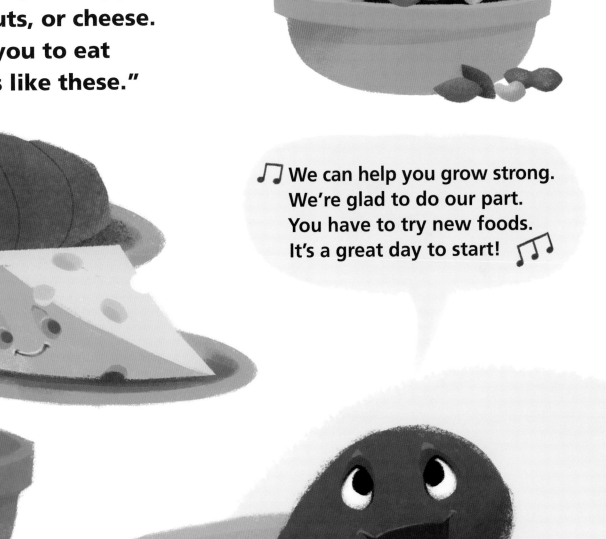

23

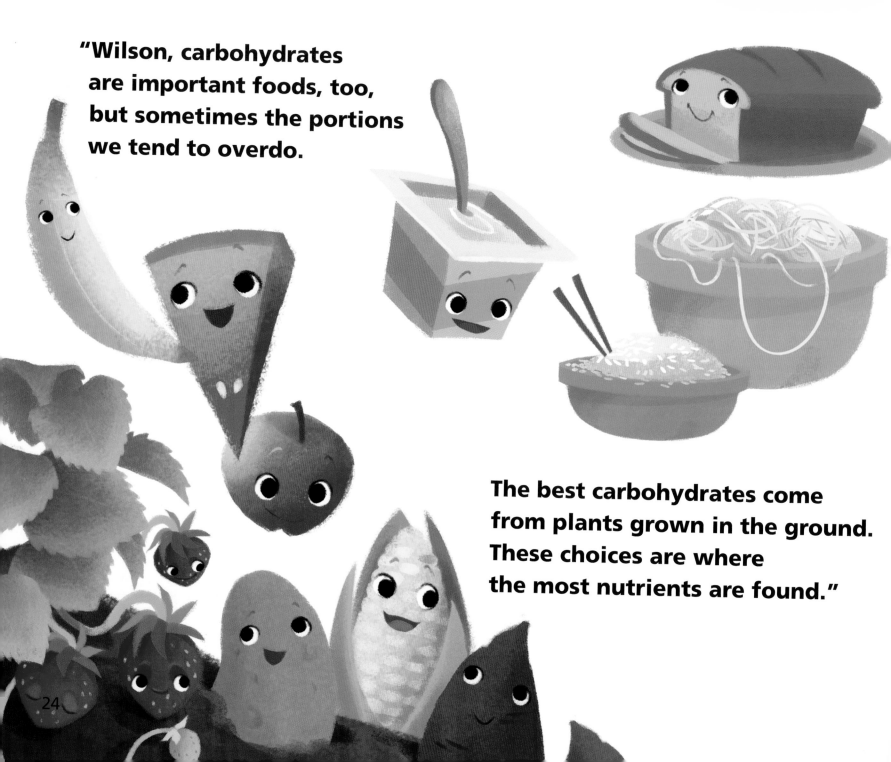

"Wilson, carbohydrates
are important foods, too,
but sometimes the portions
we tend to overdo.

The best carbohydrates come
from plants grown in the ground.
These choices are where
the most nutrients are found."

24

"This food group is the place all your sweets will fall. Remember, the key is to keep portions small."

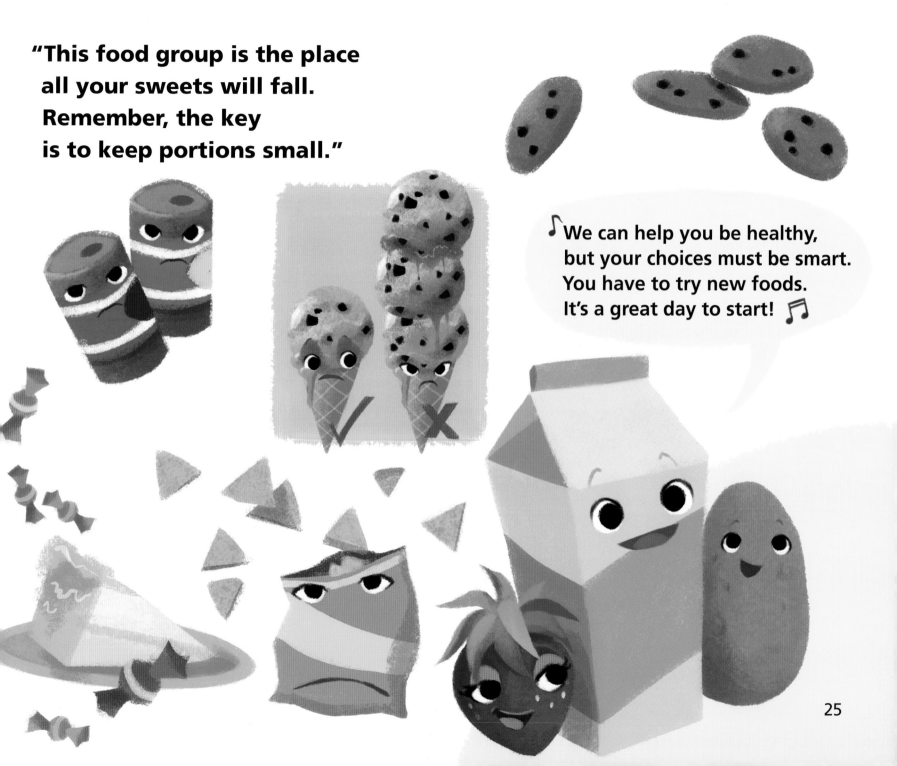

We can help you be healthy, but your choices must be smart. You have to try new foods. It's a great day to start!

**"This last food group can be misunderstood.
This group is called fats. Some are bad, some are good."**

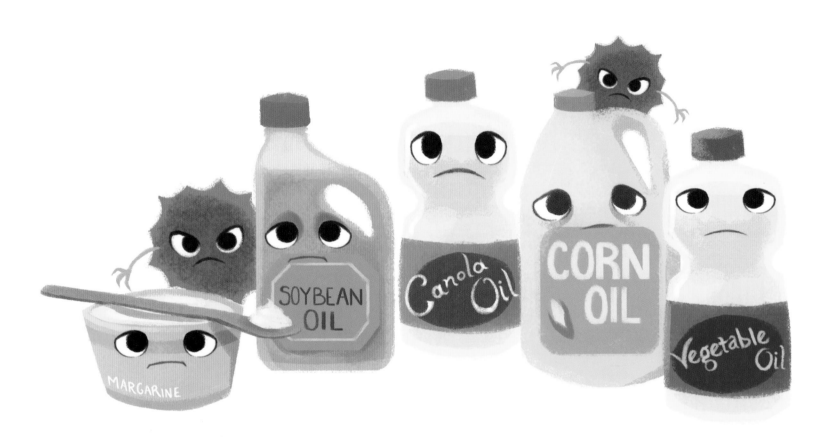

**"The healthiest fats are less processed, you see.
These are the best choices for you and for me."**

♪ Choose us, the healthy fats.
Put us in your cart.
You have to try new foods.
It's a great day to start. ♫

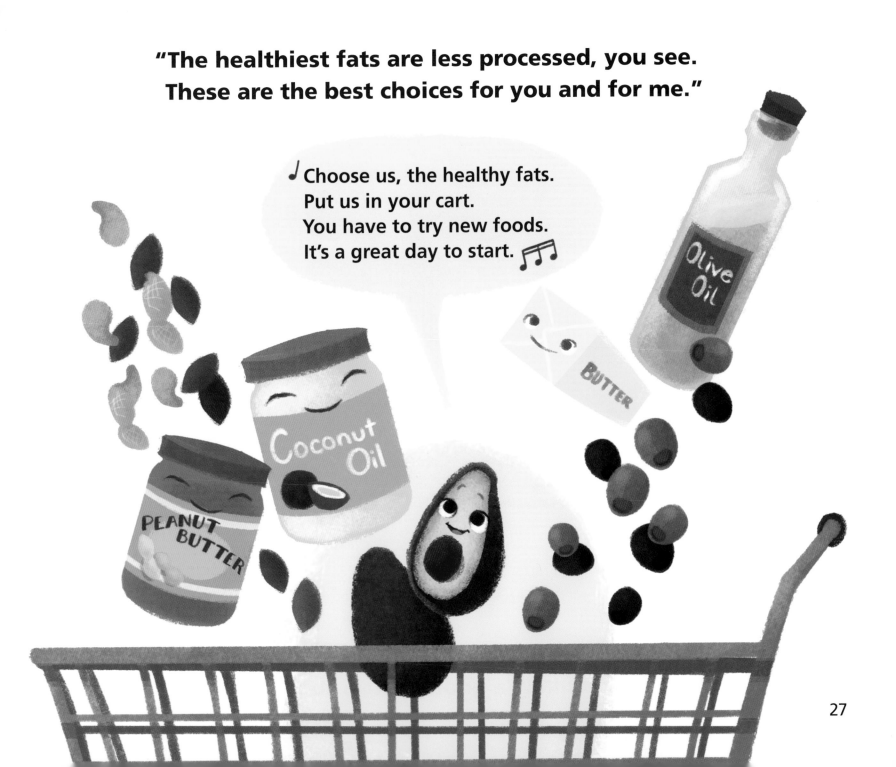

"If it's hard to decide which food is the best, just give that food the ingredients list test.

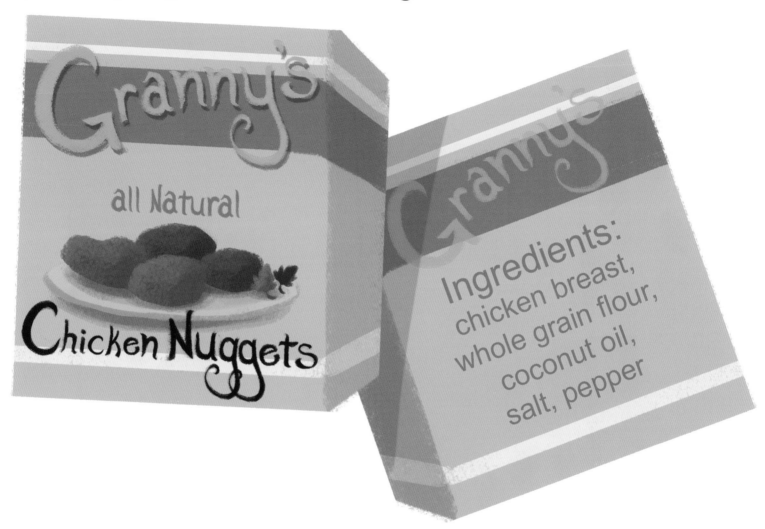

Granny's all Natural Chicken Nuggets

Ingredients: chicken breast, whole grain flour, coconut oil, salt, pepper

If the list contains mostly words that you know, that food's likely a good choice, so give it a go!"

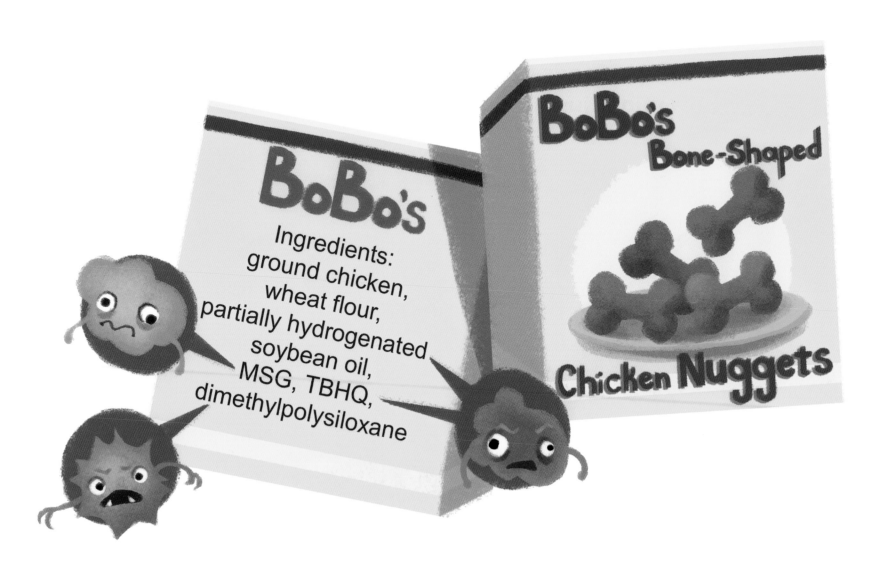

**"But if the list has words that are gobbledygoo,
who knows what that could do to you?"**

"At first, new foods might taste yucky or strange.
But you know what? Your taste buds can change!
All those foods that once tasted so crummy,
you might just find now are oh so yummy!"

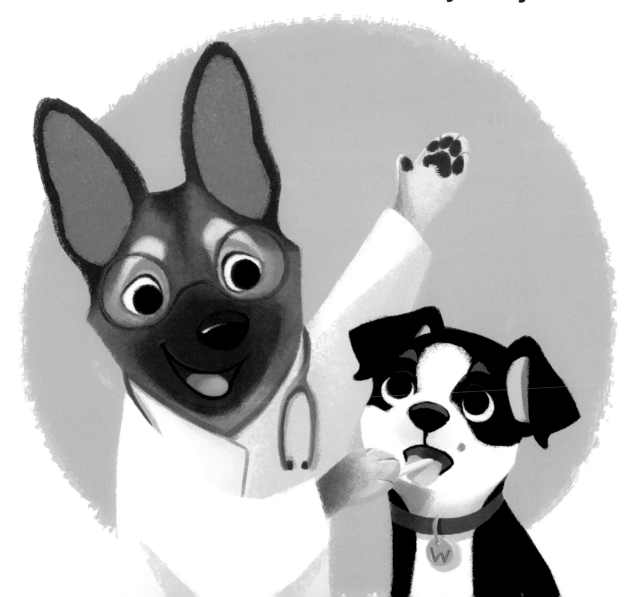

"So, my little buddy,
 these facts you now know.
 Will you eat healthy foods
 so your body can grow?"

I growled my answer,
really quiet and low.
"I just don't want to!
 I have to say no!"

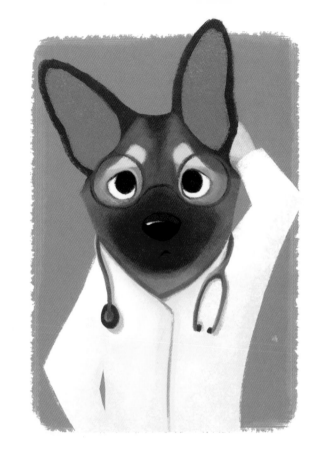

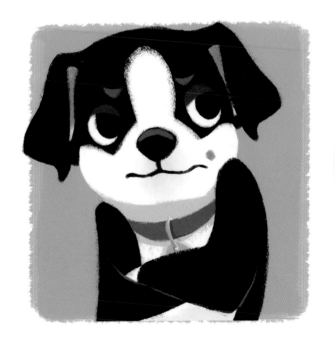

🎵 If you want to be healthy,
you need to eat smart.
You have to try new foods.
It's a great day to start! 🎵

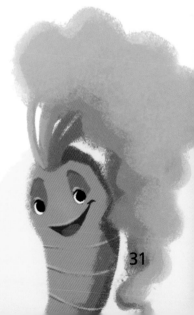

31

Mom jumped in with a bark, "Not so fast, little guy!
Being a GROUCH ON THE COUCH just WILL NOT fly!
We have to make changes, don't you see?
We'll do it together . . . the whole family!"

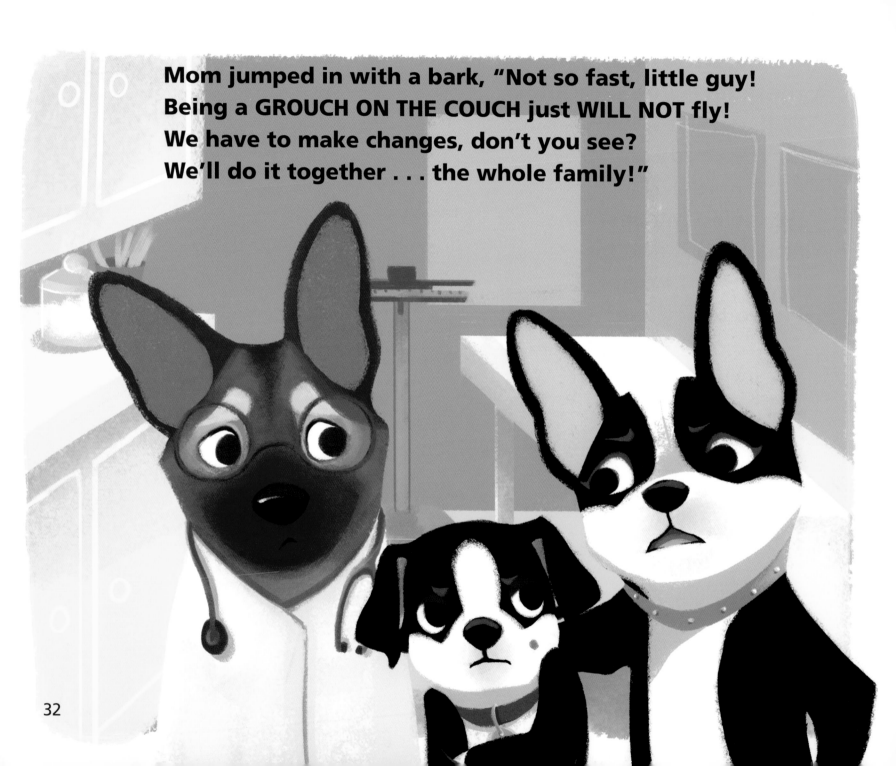

"We won't always eat right, but that's okay.
We'll just get back on board the very next day."

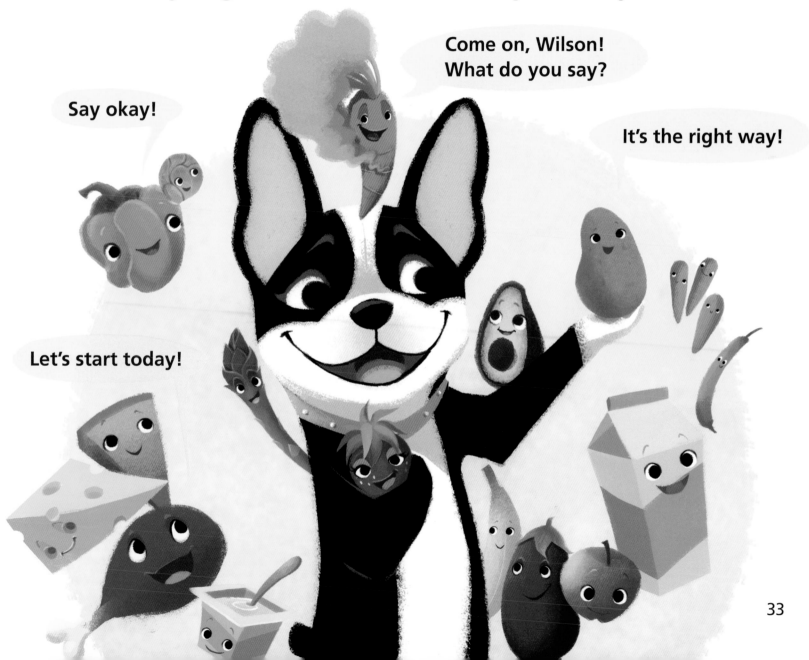

Come on, Wilson!
What do you say?

Say okay!

It's the right way!

Let's start today!

"Well, I know I'm just a kid, but I have to do my part.
I WILL try new foods! It's a great day to start!"

♩If you want to be healthy,
you need to eat smart.
You have to try new foods.
It's a great day to start! ♪

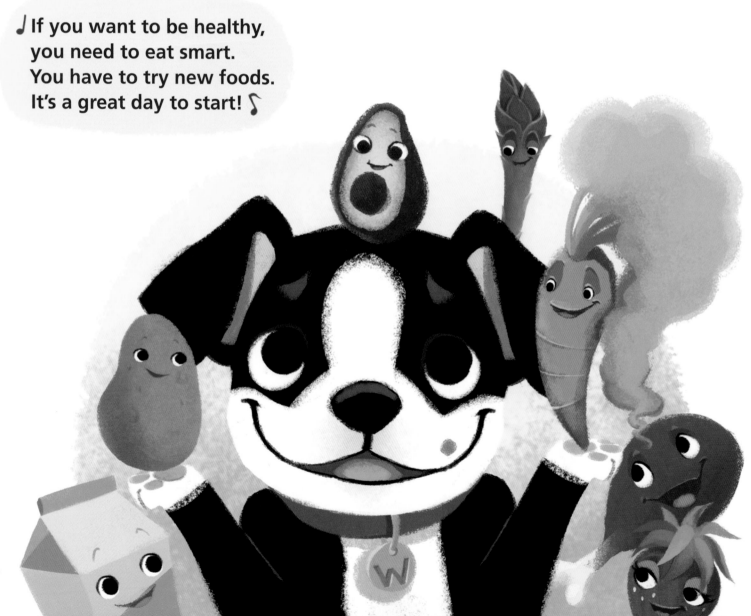

Doc hugged me and said, "I'll say no more.
Have a good time at the grocery store!"

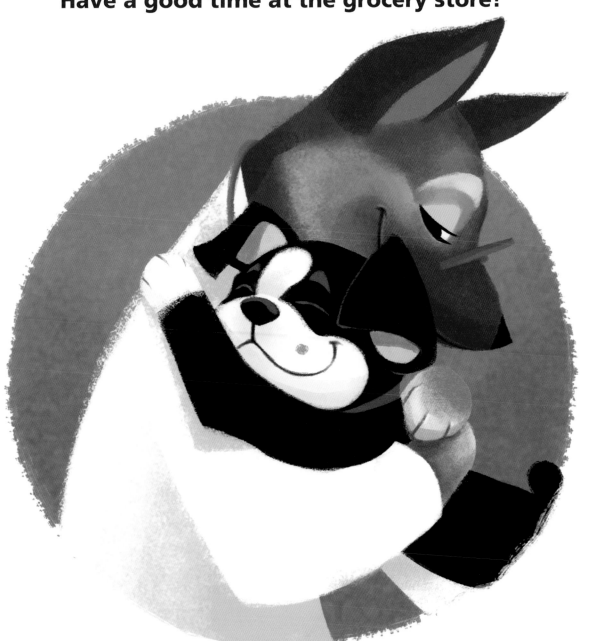

Well, it's been three months, and I have to say,
I'm trying new foods almost every day!

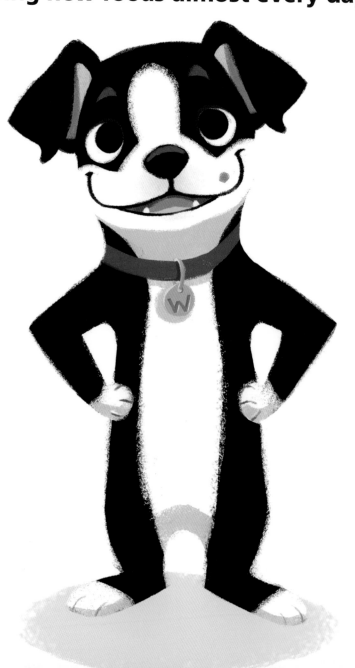

Who knew the key to being strong and smart
would begin with something like a grocery cart?

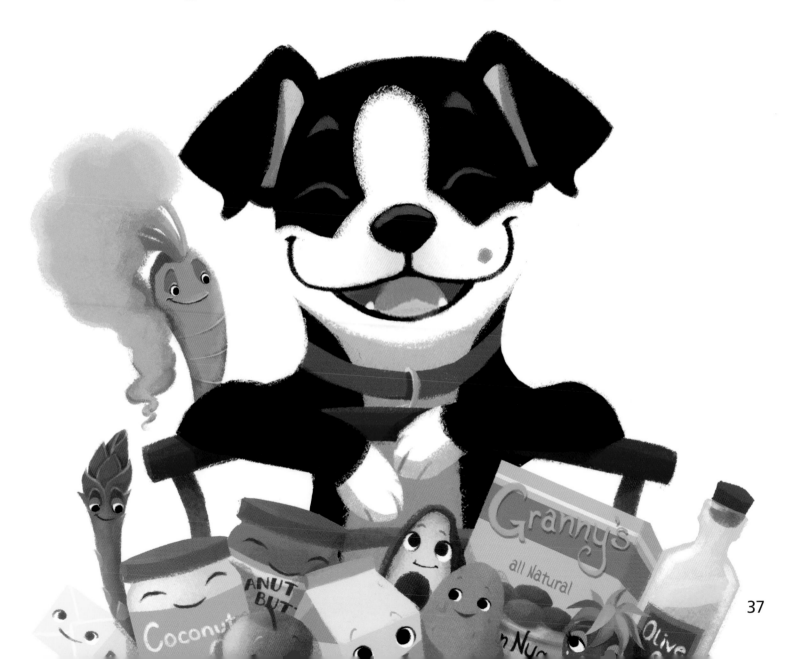

Whatever it is you love to do, eating healthy can really help you.

RUN FASTER!

JUMP HIGHER!

LEARN NEW TRICKS, TOO!

There is no limit to the things you can do!

If you want to be healthy, you need to eat smart.
You have to try new foods. It's a great day to start!

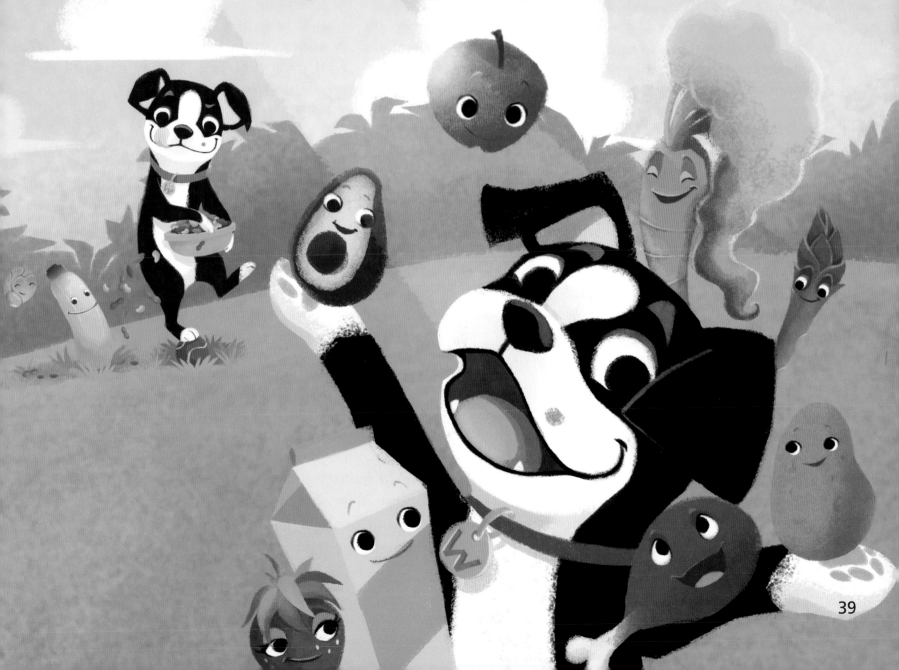

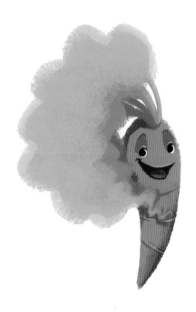

About the Author

Ashley Stewart lives in Flowery Branch, Georgia, with her husband Jay and her three children, Hadyn, Maddie, and Jack. Also living with them is the family cat, Howie, and, of course, their dog Wilson. Ashley graduated from Auburn University in 2000 with a BS in nutrition and food science. She is a registered dietitian and certified diabetes educator. Ashley enjoys teaching her family and patients about the importance of proper nutrition in achieving a healthy lifestyle. As a mother, she understands the struggle parents face trying to get their children to eat a healthy diet and try new foods. To learn more about healthy eating, visit www.EatWellWithWilson.com.

About the Illustrator

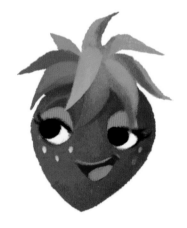

Morgan Spicer is both an animal advocate and an illustrator. Her endless love for animals, especially companion animals, can be seen through her art. She graduated from Syracuse University's BFA program in 2012 and uses her degree to educate children on the benefits of animal companionship. Morgan credits her success to her incredibly supportive family, and that includes her nine-year-old blind Shiba Inu, Kiba. She now lives and works in Manhattan with her rescue pup, Roscoe-Roo. Morgan is the founder of Bark Point Studio and aspires to open her own animal rescue and sanctuary in the future. For more information on Morgan and to see more of her work, visit www.MorganSpicerIllustration.com.